CW01151175

EATING FOR LONGEVITY

EATING FOR LONGEVITY

The Anti-Aging Diet

DECLAN HUNTER

RWG Publishing

CONTENTS

1	Introduction to Longevity and Aging	1
2	The Role of Nutrition in Longevity	4
3	Key Principles of the Anti-Aging Diet	6
4	Meal Planning for Longevity	11
5	Intermittent Fasting and Longevity	14
6	Exercise and Longevity	17
7	Stress Management and Longevity	19
8	Sleep and Longevity	21
9	Hydration and Longevity	23
10	Supplements for Longevity	25
11	The Gut Microbiome and Aging	27
12	Social Connections and Longevity	29
13	Environmental Factors and Longevity	32
14	Genetics and Longevity	34
15	Aging Gracefully: Skincare and Beauty	36
16	Mind-Body Practices for Longevity	38
17	Longevity Across the Lifespan	40

18	Longevity in Older Adults	42
19	Longevity and Chronic Disease Prevention	45
20	Culinary Techniques for Longevity	47
21	Eating for Longevity on a Budget	49
22	Ethical and Sustainable Eating for Longevity	52
23	Cultural Perspectives on Longevity and Diet	54
24	Longevity Research and Emerging Trends	57
25	Practical Tips for Incorporating Longevity Principles	59
26	Conclusion and Future Directions	62

Copyright © 2024 by Declan Hunter

All rights reserved. No part of this book may be reproduced in any manner whatsoever without written permission except in the case of brief quotations embodied in critical articles and reviews.

First Printing, 2024

CHAPTER 1

Introduction to Longevity and Aging

This idea of consuming a special diet to either avoid disease or promote a longer, healthier life is indeed the major topic of this book and a growing area of interest; people the world over are asking what they can do to slow the aging process. They start to question their own food consumption patterns and ask if there is anything to this life extension theory that seems to be ever present. More importantly, is there something that I can do such as modifying my diet that will enhance my vitality and appearance as I age? This book examines what the latest scientific evidence tells us about food and its relationship to aging and longevity. It is the purpose of this book to examine what we currently know about the relationship between food and aging, and to then modify one's diet in order to enhance one's likelihood of living a longer and healthier life.

The quest for the elusive Fountain of Youth is as old as civilization itself. Humans have been consuming special "miracle" foods and elixirs since 2000 BC in hopes that it will help restore their health, vigor, and skin to its youthful state. In the early 16th century, the Spanish explorer Ponce de Leon ventured off to The New World in search of the Fountain of Youth. Even today, thanks to Hollywood, the name given to his venture to America has been associated with "youth." Yet, twelve years later, the Spanish conquistador met his untimely death with an arrow to the leg, which became gangrenous. The concept that one can consume certain foods or, vice versa, that one can avoid certain things and live a longer, healthier life is still as popular as when Juan Ponce de Leon visited Florida.

1.1. Understanding the Science of Aging

In humans and the desire to stop the aging process, free radicals are targeted with the use of antioxidants that can stop the damage by interacting and neutralizing the free radical.

Sadly, free radicals can create unstable fatty blobs lodged along the cells that form the lining of the coronary artery, thereby beginning the plaque that causes heart disease. Free radicals can destroy protein directly, as seen in cataract formation, and can seriously damage DNA, which likely initiates the process of cancer formation. Although it is well established that the body fights free radicals wherever it can, the damage from the free radicals that escape the body's defenses may contribute to the aging process.

The free-radical theory is one of the major theories of aging. It originates from damage done to the body by free radicals, molecules containing one or more unpaired electrons. Free radicals are highly energetic and will interact with the first molecule they bump into, removing an electron from it to satisfy their unpaired condition. This action changes the victim molecule into a free radical, and the chain reaction continues until the free radicals are neutralized.

Aging at the cellular level occurs when cells overproduce defective copies of themselves, could no longer replace worn-out cells, or are prevented from moving to the area in the body where they are needed. For example, as we grow older, our skin loses its plumpness and becomes thinner and more susceptible to cuts, our hair and eyes turn gray, our reflexes become slower, and our immune responses dwindle in efficiency.

Aging is a complex and progressive accumulation of changes responsible for a wide range of effects. These changes include declining memory, impaired cognitive function, decreased immunity, organ shrinkage, reduced bone mass, muscle loss, and declining physical functions. Numerous theories have been advanced to explain the phenomenon of aging. Some researchers believe that aging is regulated by a genetically determined biological clock, while others focus on the rate of cellular growth or the cumulative buildup of cellular wastes. The truth is that the aging process is inconclusive and is the cause of extensive research by scientists.

CHAPTER 2

The Role of Nutrition in Longevity

The concept of aging is of particular interest because it occurs within a relatively narrow range throughout a species and often is accompanied by characteristic behavioral changes. Aging is defined as the process in which changes develop that increase the susceptibility of the organism to a number of diseases and impair the ability to respond to stress. The potential biological role for nutrition in retarding the aging-related processes first emerged from the studies of experimentally produced calorie restriction, which delayed the development of several age-related functional defects, such as a decrease of physiological immune responses, 32-41% of increased life spans, metabolic alterations, variations of genetic functions, and endocrine variations that can support alterations in the catabolic or anabolic processes balance in which has a role in the increase of aging. In caloric restriction, the least reactive tissues are those considered by supporting the decrease of diabetes and metabolic alterations in obese individuals compared to lean subjects.

When we think about exercise, we generally understand that it strengthens both our physical and mental health. Likewise, consuming a balanced diet composed of all the necessary nutrients and adequate energy that meets our energy needs is essential for supporting our long-term physical health. This idea of consuming the right amount of nutrients as a key to our health is clearly at the heart of the Dietary Reference Intakes used by nutrition professionals, including the Recommended Dietary Allowances and Adequate Intakes for vitamins, minerals, protein, and all other nutrients required by humans to support our long-term health. So, what role does nutrition play in longevity?

2.1. Essential Nutrients for Healthy Aging

Vitamin A, Vitamin B1, and Vitamin H help the body to release energy from carbohydrates, proteins, and fats. Vitamin B2 helps in blood formation. All of the B vitamins are important in maintaining energy and good health. Vitamin C helps the body to manufacture collagen. It helps the body heal wounds, as well as promoting healthy gums and skin. Vitamin D plays a major role in maintaining strong bones by helping the body to utilize calcium. You can get a lot of these things by eating healthy foods. Remember, what you eat can affect how you age. Eating well may help you to live longer.

Eating a diet that is rich in essential nutrients can help to protect against aging, keeping you healthy longer. Making sure that you have enough of the B vitamins, calcium, iron, and other nutrients will slow down the aging process. Vitamin C and Vitamin E actually help to defend against aging by their antioxidant powers. These vitamins help to neutralize the free radicals that are produced in the body. Free radicals can initiate disease and aging. The more of these vitamins you have, the more protection you get.

CHAPTER 3

Key Principles of the Anti-Aging Diet

3. Observe the moderate diets. Three-day diets according to P. Gory is the optimal transition to the anti-aging diet. The point is that the optimal periodicity of the diets is to achieve balance between the need of an organism in certain substances and the speed of their damage in food and in tissues where the substances route to from the alimentary canal.

2. Give preference to natural food and eat little from dainties. Dainties contain much harmful substances, including heavy metals, plasticisers, and silicone sedative, or simple dust. In general, many substances causing various diseases and influencing the vital term of the organism route into an organism with food.

1. Eat not much and a little bit less on certain days. The meal is best to be over before saturation. Stop eating when you feel that you can eat a bit more. That's the way you used to eat at childhood. And indeed, when playing much, little children often don't want to eat. As to intermittent eating that becomes recently very popular lessen eating twice a month till saturation. On these days, eat that much so that saturation would have lasted only 15 minutes and in a form of dainties.

The Anti-Aging Diet is posited to help a person live a long, healthy, and fulfilled life. When eating, it is best to observe three principal rules:

3.1. Incorporating Anti-Inflammatory Foods

Packed with vitamins C & E, experts say that including orange foods such as sweet potatoes, squash, and carrots in your diet can protect against possible skin damage and may help reverse skin aging caused by UV rays. Lycopene is a carotenoid compound found in red and pink fruits and vegetables, with it combat photo-aging and the risk for skin cancers caused by sun exposure. Pink grapefruit, watermelon, and tomatoes are all excellent sources. The healthy bacteria in probiotics can also work to keep skin supple and help slow down aging, says registered dietitian Melissa Eboli. Fermented foods like full-fat yogurt, also kefir, and sauerkraut can offer advantages against UV damage by decreasing itching and dryness.

Grappling with chronic aches, pain, and stiffness? As you age, you become susceptible to chronic inflammation, a condition that triggers unhelpful damage, characterized by higher risks of developing heart disease, cancer, diabetes, dementia, and gaining weight. Unprocessed aspects of the food you eat—think fatty fish, fresh produce—may help combat inflammatory issues by promoting your body's natural ability to regulate and repair damaged cells. On the other hand, highly processed foods, especially trans and saturated fat, the type found in greasy fried slabs and candy, may increase it.

Superfoods for Longevity

5. Spices. Spices like cinnamon, garlic, ginger, and honey are said to make a significant difference in the fight against aging. Incorporating more of these things into your diet cannot hurt.

4. Leafy greens. Leafy greens like kale, spinach, collard greens, and romaine lettuce are beneficial in the fight against aging. They are loaded with vitamins and minerals, and they are full of antioxidants too.

3. ALPHA-GPC. Chances are good that you have never even heard of alpha-glycerylphosphorylcholine before, but if you live in Italy or Spain and have dementia or other cognitive symptoms, this is a nutrient that you are already taking! It's a chemical which is released when a fatty acid found in soy and other fatty foods is broken down in the body, and it makes up a significant part of the membranes of neurons. It helps to improve cognition, or the body's ability to recognize things. Why does this matter? Because it offers the foundation of virtually all higher thought.

2. Nuts, seeds, and avocados. It has been shown that a handful of nuts a day can help to stop aging in its tracks. Eating this food can increase life expectancy and even help to maintain a healthy weight! Additionally, the monounsaturated fats in avocados have been proven to help with the actual prevention of aging.

1. Berries. Berries are a great source of fiber and can help brains stay young! Their antioxidant capacity and anti-inflammatory phytonutrients are at the heart of their anti-aging properties, and this is why we are always hearing that people should incorporate more berries into their diet in a meaningful way.

As we age, our bodies endure many changes. One thing that becomes more and more important is making sure that our diet is as supportive of good health as possible. The idea is to reduce signs of aging with a diet full of anti-aging food. If we want to grow old with grace and style, we are going to want to ensure that we are getting all of the anti-aging nutrients possible. These are some of the superfoods that are most often incorporated into an anti-aging diet.

4.1. Exploring the Benefits of Berries

In a study published in the British Journal of Nutrition, fifty-eight overweight or obese adults took seven different freeze-dried berries. The berries were: 1) strawberries; 2) raspberries; 3) blueberries; 4) blackberries; 5) cranberries; 6) black currants; and 7) lingonberries. Each berry varied in flavor and texture and contained different types and amounts of flavonoids. A high-fat, high-calorie meal was then provided. All of the berries were high in flavonoids. Blood samples were collected between 1 and 12 hours after berry consumption. Blood samples were also collected on a day when the subjects did not consume any of the study fruits, which acted as a control group. This was repeated for each of the seven berries. Several berries were found to lower postprandial insulin compared to when subjects consumed a control meal. All berries raised levels of glucagon-like peptide 1 (GLP-1) and glucose-dependent insulinotropic peptide (GIP) when compared with the control meal.

Popular and tasty berries have been receiving 21st-century attention in the nutrition and anti-aging research area. Berries are packed with antioxidants and phytonutrients that have demonstrated significant longevity benefits. Adding berries to your daily menu is as easy as sprinkling them on your morning cereal, tossing them into a blender for a lunchtime smoothie, or popping some into your mouth when you need a healthy, filling snack. The beneficial ingredients can help with heart disease, diabetes, metabolic syndrome, cancer, hypertension, memory functions, and can even reduce inflammation and liver disease. Berries contain flavonoids. These are the nutrients that give berries their color and deliver much of the expected health benefits including longevity.

CHAPTER 4

Meal Planning for Longevity

All of the foods in this diet are traditional, natural, whole foods that are high in vitamins, minerals, and phytochemicals. The only food additive that is recommended is clean, whey protein concentrate, which will help balance the amino acid profile and metabolic effects of the meals. Start your day with a breakfast that includes a mix of natural (fresh) protein at a 25-30 grams level and the right balance of complex carbs, low glycemic index, simple fresh fruit, and high potency nutritional supplement: a good multivitamin-mineral SF, a source of omega-3 EFAs, and vitamin D. The most important thing to do is make sure to make positive changes to your current diet. You don't just eat the foods that you like and that taste good to you, but rather that you are making the foods that will make it possible for your body to have a means to repair and heal itself from the inside out. Helping to keep those degenerative aging processes at significantly lower levels is your means to achieving and extending an optimal healthspan.

Meal planning for the Anti-Aging Diet is based on several principles for achieving optimum health and longevity. These include eating balanced meals made from fresh, natural, whole foods. This means you include a mix of lean protein, a wide variety of fresh vegetables and fruits (especially the cruciferous and dark leafy greens, orange-flesh squash, berries, apple, and a rainbow of other fruits and vegetables), legumes, nuts and seeds, and whole grains (we recommend primarily gluten-free whole grains, such as quinoa, brown rice, buckwheat, and amaranth, which provide a solid balance of amino acids, vitamins, minerals, and fiber). Note also that deep-sea cold water fish and clean shellfish are the best recipient sources of omega-3 EFAs for seafood eaters. Healthy fats are recommended, but in moderation, to provide the body with essential fatty acids.

5.1. Creating Balanced and Nutrient-Dense Meals

For best results, prepare meals with protein that comes from familiar and easy-to-prepare foods. If a recipe uses less than 3 ounces of a high-quality protein food such as cooked fish, meat, poultry, or tofu, make sure your portion of another side dish that contributes protein to the meal includes at least 2 tablespoons of legumes, nuts, seeds, and grains. Use the "Protein Equivalents" table to assist you in assessing the combined value of different types of protein sources in mixed meals.

While it is essential to meet your protein requirements and exceed your EAR and RDA daily, the portion size of many protein-rich cooked main dishes is large compared to the portion size planned for the other food groups on your plate. As a result, meals may become unbalanced.

Include an adequate portion of high-quality protein. Sufficient all-day protein intake in all meals will help increase your body's tolerance to stresses that occur during normal aging. Depend on primary protein sources or a combination of complete and limited amino acid protein sources.

Balance your plate. Top your plate at breakfast, lunch, or dinner with large amounts of fruits and vegetables that fill many of the colorful group plates found in this book. For optimal nutrition, fill the majority of the space on your plate. Keep in mind that dark green and orange vegetables, legumes, and starchy vegetables are very nutrient-dense, so use recipes with these foods often. Adjust serving sizes or the number of side dishes to reach the amounts necessary for desired energy and nutrient intake.

To create balanced and nutrient-dense meals, use the information and tips provided throughout this book and follow the advice to optimize protein, energy, fats, fruits, vegetables, whole grains, vitamins, minerals, and water.

CHAPTER 5

Intermittent Fasting and Longevity

So this resistance to the triggers of chronic diseases and neurodegeneration, which is beyond calorie restriction alone, is the beginning of fasting strategies on the road to a healthier and happier life. Depending on your response to intermittent fasting or your ability to carry it out, the goal of a diet-based approach is to mimic the many benefits without being overly restrictive in what you eat. One example is the 5-2 diet, where humans consume a normal diet for 5 days and two non-consecutive days consume only about 25% of their normal daily calorie intake. With many benefits that are comparable to daily prolonged fasting, alternate-day fasting can also be attempted and go for 24-36 hours without eating. Moreover, combining calorie restriction with exercise programs usually extends these benefits further. But one fact is clear: throughout multiple meals and snacks during the day and night, continuously pursuing taste, taste, and more taste could be the start of an unhealthy future.

The anti-inflammatory benefits in the brain of eating a diet with fewer calories, reductions in "bad" LDL (low-density lipoprotein-cholesterol), increases in "good" HDL (high-density lipoprotein-cholesterol), and reductions in triglycerides, fatty liver, and lower blood pressure result from the lifestyle intervention of intermittent fasting. In autophagy, which breaks down and enhances the clearance of intracellular debris, intermittent fasting also activates and stimulates the immune system. Aging is related to chronic low-grade inflammation of the brain. After only a few days of intermittent fasting, these improvements in cognitive function can be observed. And this is just the beginning as control of inflammation cascades throughout the body and reduces and manages many chronic neurodegenerative diseases. Mentally and physically, the health benefits are partially due to the cellular stress response that prepares the cells and body for the rigors of famine, making them more resilient and stronger. Control of human health outcomes appears to be under the control of present-day hunger.

A 2018 study found that people who practiced time-restricted eating saved about 8% of their energy expenditure in a day. This means that they potentially reserved more energy that was then channeled into repair and rejuvenation of cells and tissues, which is the crux of the anti-aging diet approach. Intermittent fasting is a widely used nutritional therapy for reducing the damaging consequences of aging in mammals. Many studies have demonstrated that intermittent fasting can effectively prolong lifespan while reducing mortality and morbidity in a variety of metabolic and chronic diseases.

Intermittent fasting is an eating pattern that cycles between periods of fasting and eating. It doesn't specify which foods you should eat, but rather when you should eat them. Studies have shown that it can have powerful effects on your body and brain and may even help you live longer.

6.1. The Impact of Fasting on Cellular Health

The life-extending effect of caloric restriction has attracted attention as one of the most effective methods of preventing aging. As a result, a growing number of reports suggest that fasting as an alternative approach might be quite effective as well. Although quite a few studies have linked caloric restriction to life extension, the mechanisms are still poorly understood. Nevertheless, the discovery of related genes that are evolutionarily conserved among both prokaryotes and eukaryotes provides some clues. Such a conserved gene called PNC1 was first identified in S. cerevisiae. Its mammalian counterpart was shown to participate in the function of the sirtuin family of proteins, which have NAD-dependent deacetylase activity. Such histone deacetylases are among the key players in the caloric restriction effect. Therefore, caloric restriction and fasting will be among the most promising subjects for anti-aging research in the future.

Morphological analysis of the structural changes that occur in cells in response to variations in nutrient levels has shown that chronic caloric restriction simulates the effects of famine on physiological aging. Decreasing the rate of protein synthesis elongates the lifespan of yeast cells. In fission yeast, entry into the stationary phase, which induces expression of antioxidant enzymes and activation of the stress response, occurs in response to nutrient depletion. In multicellular organisms, dietary restriction was initially identified as a factor that downregulates the hyperactivity of the insulin/insulin-like growth factor signaling pathway. This, in turn, extends the lifespan of certain model organisms including the nematode C. elegans and the fruit fly D. melanogaster. It also decreases the level of DNA damage and suppresses tumor formation in mice.

CHAPTER 6

Exercise and Longevity

Throughout the world, people who move around and get exercise live longer, healthier, and happier lives. They are leaner and have fewer degenerative age-related diseases. Exercise helps maintain participation in community and social activities, as well as sexual attractiveness and physical performance in all age groups. Among the elderly, regular physical activity helps promote weight control, relieve arthritis, lower blood pressure, improve personal appearance, promote regular bowel function, and improve blood circulation in the extremities which, in turn, retards varicose veins and hemorrhoids. The loss in aerobic fitness that accompanies aging may, however, be slowed down and partially reversed by regular exercise.

It is an a priori fact, even if there were no statistics to back it up, that people who don't exercise live shorter lives than people who do exercise. And they can expect to have some rather unpleasant diseases before they reach the end of the road. Heart disease, for example, is one of the most thoroughly researched areas of health and disease; most women think of cancer as their number-one enemy, but common or garden variety cardiovascular disease, including high blood pressure and stroke, is what brings the majority of us down in the end. Probably 85 percent or more of all heart problems are caused by what we eat and by lack of some form of physical activity.

7.1. Types of Exercise that Promote Longevity

Only specific forms of exercise are known to release IGF-I and confer the muscle anti-aging benefits. As you might guess, endurance exercise (running, swimming) is unique. The fishermen love this exercise, which actually enhances local production of IGF-1 in muscles. However, you would be wrong. That is not to say, do not run or swim because endurance exercise is well recognized for its heart anti-aging properties. However, like everything else, balance is essential. At least 20% of your muscle exercise sessions should concentrate on weight-bearing activities such as strength training. This type of exercise is consistent with improving local release of IGF-1 in muscles, which is necessary to keep our muscles age-resistant. When the IGF-I has been released locally, the effects in the long absence of other beneficial exercise are quite marked.

If you want to keep your muscles age-resistant, think about exercise. Exercise is the winning ticket in muscle stiffness because it increases the concentration of IGF-1 in muscles (compared to the rest of the body), which then travels around the body in the blood, giving essential information to stimulate virtually all areas of the body that contain muscles. Consequently, persistent use of IGF-I enhances muscle loss – great news for everybody, including older individuals concerned with their mobility and bodybuilders interested in exercise.

CHAPTER 7

Stress Management and Longevity

General stress management helps prevent physical manifestations of stress and age-related diseases. Reducing stress keeps chemical reactions in the body functioning more efficiently so that cells can repair themselves and continue to function properly. Social support in the form of a network of family and friends, increased community involvement, or mental health services is an important aspect of stress management. The ability to manage stress comes from a combination of resilience and physical and emotional health. Alter your mindset and life with relaxation techniques, meditation, expressive arts, or hobbies. These techniques are easy ways to manage stress that have a positive impact on physical and psychological health and are more powerful than frequently used coping techniques like overeating and drinking. When faced with a difficult period, turn to activities you enjoy or a close friend for stress relief.

We live in a fast-paced society where stress is a common denominator for many. Higher levels of the stress hormone cortisol tend to be correlated with negative health outcomes such as an increased incidence of age-related illnesses and a decrease in life expectancy. Fortunately, stress management is available to everyone and it is not difficult to access.

Clinical studies have shown that practices that reduce cortisol levels give us an opportunity to live a longer and healthier life.

8.1. Mindfulness Techniques for Stress Reduction

There is a great deal of confusion in contemporary America about what meditation is, so let's be a bit more specific. MBSR, in fact, uses many different kinds of meditation, as well as yoga exercises, to help people regulate the physiological processes behind stress. The major innovation of Jon Kabat-Zinn in developing the MBSR program was to take meditation out of its traditional religious or spiritual context and to translate it into American, scientific terms. While it is possible to consider the MBSR program as a form of secularized Buddhism, Kabat-Zinn has been scrupulous about removing anything from the training that smacks of dogma, even while he has remained true to the teachings in a way that is transparent to those who are interested in where these techniques originally came from.

Mindfulness-Based Stress Reduction (MBSR) is perhaps the most effective and well-documented program for treating stress. The one thing that all the other myriad stress-reduction programs seem to have in common is some form of meditation training. MBSR is a recognized and respected protocol that has been studied widely in the medical and psychological literature, and participants in the MBSR training report significant reduction in anxiety, depression, and physical symptoms related to stress, such as pain and fatigue. Researchers believe that MBSR works on many different levels to help disengage the works of the nervous system that can make stress a problem, which allows people to develop a more dispassionate attitude when dealing with the never-ending problems that life presents. MBSR enables people to operate from a platform of relaxation in stressful situations, rather than from a position of panic.

CHAPTER 8

Sleep and Longevity

Orexin is a protein that influences whether we stay asleep or wake up. Orexin also encourages calorie consumption. Age-related loss in orexin could help explain why older adults often wake up during the night, and it's possible that longer sleep influences disease chains by somehow increasing orexin, which could limit wake-up calls. Scientists are still deciphering how sleep length and orexin could be related. At one time, because longer sleep seemed to be related to longer lifespans for lab animals, some thought sleep might be one of the body's secrets to how it reverses damage. During deep sleep, the brain often handles vital repairs, and these repairs likely help decrease dangerous inflammation. The inflammation-fighting effects of sleep might be one reason it could help protect your brain with age.

While the importance of a good diet should not be minimized, nor should the importance of high-quality sleep - both are vital to promoting natural longevity and health. You should always get enough sleep, and this varies from person to person. Aging and increased inflammation can disrupt sleep and reduce sleep and REM. Studies show improved health and longevity with getting more than 7-8 hours of sleep per night. The brain cannot work against the body, so when it's deprived of sleep, it can't help us keep inflammation at bay. Sleep deprivation is inflammatory, so getting rest might be considered "anti-aging".

In animals, longer sleep is also related to less age-related brain atrophy and they have a reduced risk of death.

9.1. The Importance of Quality Sleep for Anti-Aging

The ability to accumulate this work while maintaining adequate rest and relaxation is critically important for all of us. I maintain that a lower chronic disease rate equals either a longer healthspan or lifespan, which equals a greater wellnessspan. Thus, one can hypothesize that the quality and quantity of a necessary amount of sleep leading to less insulin resistance leads to an enhanced ability to focus and concentrate leads to a corresponding increase in the individual's productivity at work. In addition, adhering to an anti-aging strategy leads to an improved ability to be fully present in all aspects of life: being truly present with myself, really with our loved ones, and really with our environment. I would argue that looking at the long game, this would have suggested to many of us that we become more mindful about how we manage and live our lives.

By now, the picture is overwhelming that in terms of getting in a natural weight, in terms of getting less depressed, in terms of improving your memory and helping to fight against dementia, and in terms of overall vitality, getting a minimum of seven hours of sleep per night linked to less chronic disease. We live in a 24/7 world. Fifty years ago we did not have data to know that we should be exercising 30 minutes a day or a minimum of 10,000 steps a day. Fifty years ago we did not have the data telling us that we should avoid trans fats and non-caloric sweeteners. Fifty years ago we did not have data saying that if you get less than six or seven or eight or sometimes nine hours of sleep at night, your overall chronic disease rate is much higher. If you get a good night's sleep, you are going to have a better wakeful time, and that wellness is going to last longer.

CHAPTER 9

Hydration and Longevity

Water requirements vary according to a number of factors, but a good rule of thumb is to aim to drink five to six 8- to 10-ounce glasses of filtered, purified water every day. Drinking at least one glass before meals helps fill your stomach and supports weight-loss efforts. And if you're relying instead on unnecessary calories from sugary beverages, drinking water instead can help you lose about 5 pounds in a year. What's more, drinking water and other calorie-free beverages instead of other drinks that contain sugar is associated with a lower risk of developing heart disease. Drink water, green tea, or another non-caloric beverage instead of a high-calorie, high-sugar or high-fat beverage.

Making sure you're drinking enough water to stay well-hydrated during the day is a fundamental part of living the Anti-Inflammation Diet lifestyle and contributing to your optimal health and longevity. You need to keep your body well-hydrated so it can function at an optimal level. Every one of your cells is suspended in water, kind of like the meat in a watermelon. The more easily water can move into and out of cells, the more efficiently your body can function to perform all the physiological activities required for health and well-being, including detoxification.

10.1. Benefits of Proper Hydration for Aging Well

The basic principles of the "Tao of Longevity" Anti-Aging Program involve learning about healthful food preparation, food combining, and learning to make wise eating choices. Our nutritional guidelines also depend on the proper intake of necessary vitamins, minerals, and essential nutrients and daily hydration with pure water, fresh juices, green tea, and other healthful beverages. The "Tao of Longevity" Anti-Aging Program focuses on fresh, organically grown fruits, vegetables, and leafy greens. Wild foods, nuts, seeds, whole cooked grains, and cooked or raw seafood and suitable poultry are also included in an excellent diet program. Since ancient times, these food and beverage guidelines have consistently produced the best longevity results for people living in the Blue Zone regions of our planet, as well as for generations of the longest-lived old men and women in the world. Now, you can use our new and innovative tools, tips, and delicious recipes to help you look and feel your best your whole life.

Welcome to the "Tao of Longevity" website and our anti-aging lifestyle program, which you can adopt to enjoy better health, happiness, and longevity your whole life! On our site, you can learn about the latest scientific advances and ancient secrets for healthful living. Plus, you can begin (by making easy positive changes one step at a time) a new and healthier way of eating and drinking. You will learn about the ancient "Tao" secret of living happier, longer, and better! Our personal anti-aging nutrition program does not involve any drugs, pills, super potions, shots, treatments, personal care products, or surgery.

CHAPTER 10

Supplements for Longevity

Starting around age forty, women need to boost calcium intake and men may also need to do so. Our body's ability to absorb calcium decreases with age. Thirst often decreases, making it easy to drink less and eat less, and therefore calcium intake also decreases. Take at least 600 mg of calcium twice a day. In addition, take 400 to 800 IU of vitamin D in a supplement plus food or beverage in the diet that is vitamin D fortified. Get plenty of foods rich in vitamin D at the same time, like cheese and milk with vitamin D in it, liver, meat, and concentrated food sources of vitamin D, such as fatty salt-water fish like herring or salmon, eggs from chickens fed vitamin D, and sunlight to make the body produce vitamin D.

No one's diet, no matter how healthful, can meet all the body's needs for vital nutrients after about age thirty. That's when supplements must start bridging the gap between what a person should take in and what they actually do. Knowing what to take can add a lot of good years to a person's life. Here are the supplements that are good buys in several ways: they're safe, they often make a difference in a person's life, and they are also cheap.

11.1. Evidence-Based Supplements for Anti-Aging

When the supplements in this program are taken long-term with specific diet and exercise strategies, there is significant potential to slow the aging process and substantially extend the human lifespan. Although much of the anti-aging community looks forward to more powerful life extension and anti-aging therapies coming in future decades, in 2008, there is only mainstream scientific and medical data to evaluate the potential effectiveness of life-extending dietary supplements. While there are many other supplements that do present significant potential to slow aging beyond currently available life-extension medication, there is less evidence - high quality, innovative, and costly scientific studies in humans - on which to make confident predictions, in the judgment of scientists and clinicians focused on the aging process and role in biology. These key therapies could become part of a specialized, life-extending therapy in future decades.

Currently, no dietary supplements guarantee a longer life, and none can turn back aging - no matter their reputation. However, substantial evidence from over 75 years of high-quality research suggests that certain supplements can directly target the aging process. Especially powerful at slowing aging are the use of a combination of the common supplements, sometimes used in specialized formulations designed to fight the aging process. These are the most potent supplements that science now offers to extend life, maximize mental clarity, lead a productive and enjoyable life, maintain a youthful sex drive, and avoid chronic diseases, including many types of cancer, and the number one killer of the Western world, cardiovascular disease (CVD).

CHAPTER 11

The Gut Microbiome and Aging

So, in considering the gut as an organ strongly involved in overall health maintenance, vegetable food intake would seem to be a beneficial key factor. Indeed, several studies have shown that eating vegetarian food can help to maintain the bacterial diversity of the gut throughout life. Moreover, the gut microbiota seems also to be responsible for the observed differences: the ingestion of L-carnitine, L-carnitine-containing food, and choline, which are present in animal food and particularly in red meat, favors the presence of bacteria which produce trimethylamine N-oxide from the presence of choline related or L-carnitine related, promoting disease.

Our understanding of the importance of the microbes that live in our gut has significantly increased in the last 10 or so years. The gut microbiome, the collection of all the microbes in the gut, has been linked to many important functions in the body such as metabolism, immune function, and brain health. Conversely, disturbances of the gut microbiome have been linked to many aging-related diseases. These diseases are not only localized to the gut but can have effects throughout the body and brain. Treatment of the gut with probiotics, fecal transplants, and changes in diet can have a huge impact on the progression of conditions like depression, Parkinson's disease, obesity, diabetes, cardiovascular disease, many kinds of neurological symptoms such as sleeping and epilepsy, and many gastrointestinal diseases.

12.1. Understanding the Role of Gut Health in Longevity

The beneficial effects of eating the whole plant are largely due to the fact that plant compounds from fruits, vegetables, and whole grains can pass through our system without being absorbed or digested. These ingredients can at the same time help to nourish our internal bacterial community by fermenting the indigestible carbohydrates that the friendly bacteria love into various strains of Bifidobacteria. These fermented ingredients can lower our circulating cholesterol levels, and at the same time improve our glucose metabolism. In addition, probiotics can help us to break down plant phenolic compounds into smaller molecules that are absorbed into our systems. These bioactive molecules have antioxidant effects, and in some cases may also work to help turn genes involved in our body's defense against inflammation and cancer on, or off.

When we're looking at healthy aging, another area we should explore is our gut. This inner tube of ours plays many important roles whether we are two years old or one hundred years old. What we eat and drink serves as the "assembly line" for remaking us. Synthesizing the body's cells and tissues with the 45 known nutrients, 53 minerals, 18 amino acids, and ~13 vitamins require good digestion and a complex interaction of a diverse microbial colony that resides in our GI tract. Abundant and diverse bacterial populations in the GI tract co-exist with the 90-95% of cells that are in there to assist "us" in the digestive process. All of these little "helpers" make it possible for our cells and tissues to regenerate as needed, keeping our energy up and our immune defenses ready. But in addition to working with us to make sure we are working at our most efficient, this large and abundant microbiota community has much more to do with anti-aging health. People with a diverse community of friendly bacteria in their gastrointestinal (GI) tract seem better able to maintain a healthy weight and are less likely to be obese. These people also have less inflammation and other metabolic problems.

CHAPTER 12

Social Connections and Longevity

Spending time with friends also may help promote good health. Every time you get together, you're likely to share stories, laughter, encouragement, advice, and support. Positive, happy people have a contagious effect on others, even to the extent they are helpful in preventing the onset of the common cold. Whether we are in person or connecting through social networking, we are supporting each other in making diet and healthful lifestyle decisions. Behaving in such an upbeat manner is a simple, yet effective, way to improve health and longevity. If you share the contents of this book, any of the Mary's Mini-Meal Plans, and the accompanying recipes, with family and friends, you are providing free, healthful gifts of love.

Isolation can reduce quality and quantity of life. People with limited social connections are more likely to die earlier after a heart attack or cancer diagnosis than similar ones with larger networks. Sometimes, there aren't any nearby community or religious groups to join. In such case, there is always a solution: make new friends. As you meet people and share your interests, hobbies, talents, war stories, help out where needed, learn a new skill, create something beautiful, or get involved in a cause bigger than yourself, your health and happiness will both benefit. It's always possible to widen your social circle and transform acquaintances into cherished friends.

Numerous research studies have confirmed that enjoying a network of social connections can promote health and longevity. A happy marriage is associated with longer life. Family and friends are important too. People with strong connections have reduced stress, improved motivation to care for themselves, improved immune function, and lower risk for chronic diseases such as cancer and heart disease.

13.1. Impact of Relationships on Aging Well

Margaret L. Warthinger found that relationships can be important until the very end of life. In a large study of people over 50, Warthinger surveyed the widowed and discovered that friends were the most important people in terms of remaining active, interested, and happy. Even new friends diminished the sadness and loneliness experienced by the displaced spouse. These findings concur with the Harvard study directed by George Valliant—connectiveness is important to age successfully. As Warthinger writes, "This lasting preference for more personal interactions reflects the enduring nature of personal relationships as buffers against the losses entailed in disruption of the marital bond." With all of the advances science has made, social connectedness is also a way to help slow the aging process. When you connect to others, your brain also stays younger. Why is it that relationships can have a positive impact on the aging brain? One reason is the beneficial health effects and fewer neurotic habits that are associated with relationships. Within the family context, the benefit is greatest with the spouse or partner, and the beneficial neurological effects decrease as you move farther away from the spouse, according to the study conducted by Audrey N. Samson and her team.

Connections are important to aging well. As George Vaillant describes, "Successful aging is about the interactive effects of all aspects of the self in relation to the self, the environment, and the person whom one has become." Vaillant, who directed the long-term Harvard longitudinal study, discovered that relationships play a major role in well-being.

In fact, of the seven major factors his research uncovered, five are connected to relationships: physical activity, emotional avoidance, adaptive coping style, absence of depression, and alcohol abstinence. The other two factors are the number of years in school and smoking cessation. The good news is that we can maintain friendships. Others who have studied aging populations have reached similar conclusions. George E. Valliant, Aging Well: Surprising Guideposts to a Happier Life from the Landmark Study of Adult Development (New York: Little, Brown, 2002).

CHAPTER 13

Environmental Factors and Longevity

The Eating for Longevity Way: The Anti-Aging Diet has the following recommendations to offer for environmental sources: Eat a variety of foods to ensure that you get all the nutrients necessary to combat aging. There is no secret food; eating for longevity requires a variety of nutrients that act together in complex ways that are beyond our understanding. Eat foods that meet U.S. Dietary Guidelines. Although these guidelines don't take into account all the nutrients lacking in today's foods, the guidelines offer a valuable starting point for determining good general eating guidelines. Eat carefully. Many environmental toxins come hidden within the foods you eat.

Unfortunately, you can eat the healthiest diet imaginable and succumb to environmental hazards such as a bridge collapse. But, your diet can help prevent or minimize many of the environmental factors that threaten your life span. For example, free radicals, the most prevalent environmental problem, usually result from environmental pollutants. Getting your antioxidants from your diet can reduce much of the damage from these pollutants. The next section highlights some environmental problems that can either be prevented or minimized by getting nutrients from your diet.

14.1. Avoiding Toxins and Pollutants for Healthy Aging

Pesticides, insecticides, and herbicides are powerful oxidizing chemicals because they damage small organisms and harm plant life. Soaps, detergents, and shampoos are oxidizing chemicals that disrupt the fatty layers in the hair and skin. Phase one and phase three of the detoxification system can produce poisonous components when pollutants are acted on to salvage them from harming the cell. Oxygen is an oxidizing nutrient when indirectly converted to toxic and poisonous forms in the cells. Chlorine is a skin and lung irritant when inhaled or eaten in baked or canned products. Some drugs and anesthetics can convert healthier nutrients to poor and degraded components. Small doses of food additives and drinking water disinfection chemicals can be toxic and deadly when overdosed or over-ingested. To avoid these harmful chemicals and their toxic effects, detoxification is necessary to maintain good health and prevent premature aging of the human body.

Each and every cell in our body has to be protected from oxidative chemicals in the body. Air pollution, water pollution, and UV rays from the sun produce chemicals that are inhaled or ingested into the body. These chemicals are called free radicals, and they are oxidizing chemicals that can damage cells. Pollutants that are oxidizing and injurious to the cells internally are produced from nitric oxide, hydrogen peroxide, peroxynitrite, hypochlorite, hypobromite, hypochlorous acid, lipid hydroperoxides, hydroxyl radicals, superoxide, singlet oxygen, and peroxyl radicals. These chemicals are all highly reactive and can destroy all components of a human cell, including lipids, proteins, and DNA.

CHAPTER 14

Genetics and Longevity

In order to affect whether or not you age quickly or slowly, a gene does not necessarily have to change or even to be defective, but it does have to be expressed and active in a certain way - and that regulation is influenced over one's lifetime by diet. Studies show that during aging, there is an increase in oxidative damage and a decrease in the function of proteins that repair that damage and often of proteins themselves. Yet, increasing the expression of these antioxidant enzymes improves longevity. Similarly, a reduction in the incidence of age-related heart disease and stroke occurs when a specific gene that contributes to an age-related increase in inflammation is turned off. Furthermore, when resistant proteins are increased in animals, they generate more resistance to environmental stresses and live much longer lives.

In addition to engineering foods, there's a growing body of research aimed at designing drugs to help maintain an organism's natural vitality - ideally causing a person to remain relatively healthy throughout a longer lifespan. In fact, advertisers make money on nearly every newsstand promising what the aged have longed for throughout human history: a way to stop the clock on the aging process. This is the science of biogerontology, and while it focuses mainly on the genes and cellular pathways involved in aging and might ultimately make cosmetic and much healthier lifespans a reality, it has a side effect of altering the caloric processing and metabolic pathways, making the aging process and its effect on longevity a bit more manageable than through dietary restriction alone.

15.1. Exploring the Genetics of Aging

The aging process is most obviously identified upon observing external changes beneath the skin. Unseen but more vital are the internal changes affecting every living cell. These cellular changes progress in a person's body, possibly pushing the balance of disease or health. Biologists have identified and characterized a number of genes speculated as key players in the aging process. They have a great passion for aging research, being arguably the most elusive questions in biology. To make the problem more exciting, aging is the greatest single risk factor for a wide variety of chronic diseases. Reasoning indicates that, by extending the human lifetime average, we are also likely to delay the onset of the most prevalent of these diseases.

When we look at a photograph of someone in old age, we see a face etched with the history of the person's life, which may include good nutrition, extensive exercise, and a never-ending parade of vitamins, herbs, and supplements. Or a life of smoking, little exercise, and a steady diet of trashy novels and cookies. Or the coin toss of nearly opposite health histories. At age 60 and beyond, our DNA may be able to mask good or bad living. Our genes may appear identical, but their levels of expression vary from person to person, making each of us genetically unique and susceptible to different chronic diseases from other people. And so each transparent landscape of fine lines, hidden beneath a weathered face, yields hints as to our genetic legacy.

CHAPTER 15

Aging Gracefully: Skincare and Beauty

Frequent consumption of antioxidants is the best strategy for preventing cosmetic and other surgery and protecting the skin from ultraviolet-induced damage and photo-aging. Healthy, growing skin demands an ample supply of powerful opposing antioxidants that neutralize free radicals and allows normal skin function. Granules, a fat-soluble carotenoids, are important constituents of the human diet, known for their excellent antioxidant activity and ability to protect the skin from UV-induced oxidative stress. According to the British Society for Nutrition, scientists in the UK have shown that women of a healthy life diet group who ate 2.5 tablespoons sun-dried tomatoes and 10 grams olive oil per day for 3 months could decrease the number of UV-induced skin burning cells and DNA damage. Overall, tomatoes are beneficial antioxidants. Because antioxidants quench oxidation by giving up part of themselves to ensure that the body stays healthy, consuming 6 to 10 tomatoes per week is recommended.

One of the most potent antioxidants and anti-inflammatory agents is glutathione, and because of its skin-rejuvenating properties, glutathione is usually delivered in high doses for beauty and anti-wrinkle effect. Glutathione is also protective against the invasion of a foreign body or harmful microorganism, bacteria, or virus. When the human body is under stress, sick, or near the end of its life, glutathione becomes so low in the bloodstream that if the pathogen attempts to invade, there is not enough line of players to stop the bacterial invasion. This is the time when the human body shuts down immune function and loses the ability to make the disease-fighting bacterial patrol. Moreover, synthetic compounds can only provide a temporary effect and can be harmful to the organ function if taken over the recommended dosage, but still many people want a quick skincare or beauty effect and use it anyway.

16.1. Natural Skincare Tips for Anti-Aging

Another tip is argan oil, which is frequently known as Moroccan oil. This natural skincare is very good for your skin, especially for a number of reasons. Argan oil is very rich in antioxidants, unsaturated fatty acids and is naturally rich in vitamins to increase the potential of anti-aging. Researchers found that the oil combined with other vitamins has anti-aging advantages. Pine and coconut oils can work wonders as the best natural skincare. None of these solutions come from the chemists, only from the best of nature. Since there are no artificial preservatives added to the mix, the vitamins are quickly absorbed by the lower skin layers and provide the nutrients necessary to help the skin.

The search for natural skincare tips for anti-aging has been on for a long time. There are a lot of ideas out there. Some of them are good, but you cannot use them all. These natural skincare tips will have you on your way to healthy, beautiful skin. Start with a diet rich in fiber to help get rid of toxins. Omega-3 fatty acids can give you the best skin that you have ever had. Healthy fats can help with your diet. A good source of healthy fat comes from fish. This can help your skin look younger. Almonds are a good source of antioxidants. These natural skincare tips are aimed at keeping you and your skin looking younger until you are very old.

CHAPTER 16

Mind-Body Practices for Longevity

You will greatly benefit from the use of mind-body techniques. By activating and nurturing the divine through meditation, you could even make the changes in only a week. Meditation can help heal emotionally and spiritually, and Chi Kung can take care of the side of internal exercises. These side effects include the beauty benefits associated with longevity. Balancing alone can create an effect akin to cosmetic surgery and chemical beautifiers. Adopting a mind-body lifestyle can help both your appearance and longevity, all without the need for drug therapy or surgery.

Simply treating your body with care is not enough for a long, vibrant life. You need a mind that is equally healthy. You can create an atmosphere for cultivating your mind with internal practices, such as qigong, tai chi, or yoga. These ancient approaches to mental and physical health can naturally and effectively charge you with youthfulness. Internal cultivation creates an energetic field designed specifically for perpetual youth, boosting your heart's energy, enhancing the brain's functioning, and improving the circulation, balance, and processing of nourishing and cleansing fluids and qi. Such fluid balance creates youthful skin, hair, and vision.

17.1. Yoga and Meditation for Healthy Aging

Yoga is also shown to build muscle tone and sheath the body in lean muscle, imparting strength without bulkiness. Yoga also promotes muscle relaxation that can reduce age-related stiffness and pain associated with other fitness routines. In addition to building muscle strength and muscle tone, yoga also tones and massages soft internal organs, facilitating good circulation. Yoga's strengthening, stretching, and massaging actions help every organ, gland, blood vessel, and muscle in the body move—and move properly. This helps transport blood containing plenty of life-giving oxygen to the cells so that the "moderately active" portion of their energy needs can be fueled efficiently, rejuvenating not just the physical body, but the mind and spirit.

Most people believe yoga is about toning the body and reducing stress. But scientific evidence is proving that regular practice of yoga can indeed slow down the aging process. In a recent German study, practicing yoga was found to affect the rate of telomere loss, potentially keeping skin and organs young. Another study showed that practicing yoga and meditation can help in reducing oxidative stress and inflammation at the cellular level. Considered the "measure of biological aging," oxidative stress can cause the aging shifts due to DNA, cell deterioration, and loss of skin elasticity and muscle tone.

CHAPTER 17

Longevity Across the Lifespan

The major causes of reduced function or premature death of many older adults—atherosclerosis, cancer, diabetes, dementia, osteoporosis, and arthritis—can be delayed, or in some cases completely prevented, through healthful nutrition, moderate physical activity, and absence of tobacco use. In Chapter 1, we focused on the optimal diet, one that is rich in natural plant foods, and the relationship between this dietary pattern and an increased number of years between life and death. In this chapter, we'll look more directly at the aging process per se. First, we define this process and then explore the relationships between nutrition, health, and behavior as they pertain to successful aging. Finally, we'll discuss the evidence for the ability of nutrition to influence aging, specifically the relationship between calorie intake and longevity and the association between dietary practices and chronic disease prevention.

Although maximal life span is determined by the genetic messages that program the molecular processes that underlie aging, a healthy life is within the grasp of most people who have access to good health care. Successful aging means maintaining a high level of physical and mental function well into the later years, ideally until death. No one really wants to live, no matter what it means to be old. Individuals can take charge of their own aging process by adopting a firm commitment to making the right healthy lifestyle choices in relation to diet, physical activity, and dietary supplement use.

18.1. Promoting Longevity in Children and Adolescents

Good health is based on many factors and diet is fundamental to long-term health, but there are additional considerations to longevity. Air and manual pollution, ultraviolet damage from the sun, dangerous working conditions, and living in high-crime neighborhoods, all contribute to premature aging. Significant increases in lifetimes made through medical intervention urge increased research on anti-aging nutrition in order to assure higher productivity and freedom from chronic diseases. With nutrition-related health care costs on the rise, the increasing longevity of the population is assuming significant proportion and many of the elderly people are in good health. This is making anti-aging nutrition an important health issue for the future of our country.

The search for an anti-aging diet is not limited to adults but begins with good nutrition in childhood. Remarkable strides have been made in extending the lifespan of people of all ages through modern medicine and surgery, but no surgery or miracle medical discovery is more powerful than teaching our children the life-extending power of a healthful, nutritious diet. It is estimated that 30 percent of all cancer deaths are caused by dietary factors, while other nutritionally related diseases, such as heart disease, hypertension, and stroke, account for a large portion of our health care expenditures. Replacement of nutrient-deficient, calorie-dense foods (those high in saturated fats, sugar, and glycerides, etc.) in the early years will provide the energy needed for mental and physical activity, and will lay the foundation for health and longevity in older years.

CHAPTER 18

Longevity in Older Adults

Important links between energy, health, and optimal aging indicate a special requirement of more energy to support the aging process. A lower financial status explains, in part, some of the malnutrition in elderly people, as well as the decreased need for food and low food preferences or inadequate food preparation. Simple changes in nutrient and meal plans will not mitigate the issue of hunger and malnutrition. However, such changes provide a starting point for symptoms such as delayed wound healing, reduced muscle mass, poor appetite, and certain nutrient deficiencies, which can result in malnutrition in elderly individuals if left unnoticed. Such dietary changes might include frequent meals and snacking, as well as improved meal nutritional quality.

The majority of people reaching old age want to live in good health and maintain a certain quality of life until they die. In other words, people do not only aspire to live a long life but also aim to sustain their mental and bodily function, social participation, and meaningfulness in living as long as possible. A key element of the ability of elders to maintain a certain mental and physical quality of life emerges from their nutritional status, with numerous age-related changes that affect the nutritional state. Decreased energy needs, associated with decreased physical activity and the negative implications of an incorrect diet on the health of aging individuals, are some of the chief challenges of being elderly. Older adults require proper nutrition and sufficient energy intake, but how much energy is required varies from individual to individual.

The process of becoming older involves biological (genetic, molecular, cellular, etc.), psychological (mental, cognitive, etc.), and social (societal, cultural, etc.) elements. Even in late life when biological processes are contributors to physical and mental decline, older adults project a high degree of contentment with their life, despite ongoing age-related changes such as declining health, loss of social and financial resources, and the death of their loved ones. The mode of thinking about old age has changed dramatically in recent times, with more and more people entering the physical age of old age. Perceptions about healthy nutrition in old age have altered, as now more than ever, aging is associated with possibilities, new ideas, experiences, and vitality. The promotion of healthy aging is becoming a major challenge and task for all societies around the world. Increased life expectancies and a reduction in birthrates in various societal regions have led to an increasing number of elderly people with a decrease in the ratio of young to old people within communities.

19.1. Strategies for Healthy Aging in Seniors

We should also ensure that we have good reserves of important nutrients such as calcium, vitamins D and K, etc. Although age is considered unchangeable, chronological age is somewhat deceiving as it is the time someone has existed on this planet. It does not consider important differences inside the body. These variations, the easier to change of the two types of age, account for the majority of high-quality life's available time. As we age, the later-life changes that take place inside our body and that increase the chance of ill health and early mortality are also experienced by all our friends and counterparts. They are influenced by their body composition, poor nutritional status, mode of nutrition and well-being, or a generally less healthy lifestyle and level of well-being. Our body's response to a better diet and increased physical activity is still feasible and reversible even in later life. This should be welcomed as we are now living longer and enjoying our later years more than before. In contrast, having to endure a life in a state of physical purity is unattractive.

A positive, flexible approach to advancing years, in conjunction with a supportive lifestyle and diet, provides the best chance for a healthy, extended life. Aging is considered in terms of a number of significant issues that arise in older age including bone health, immunity and inflammation, and memory and cognition. The great news is that late-life changes can still be significantly modified by changes in diet and lifestyle. The increased chronic, nonlethal diseases like hypertension, coronary heart disease, cardiovascular disease, type 2 diabetes, chronic inflammation, and immune deficiency caused by poor diet seem to increase with age. As a general rule, to reduce the damage caused by inflammation and immune deficiency as we age, we need to reduce our intake of saturated and trans fatty acids and high-glycemic-load foods and ensure good intake of omega-3 fatty acids, fiber-rich foods, and fruit and vegetables.

CHAPTER 19

Longevity and Chronic Disease Prevention

It is known that nutrition affects growth, development, function, reproduction, and maintenance of the human body on a day-by-day basis for life, as does medicine. Therefore, it is important to consume a meal that includes food containing essential nutrients to maintain good health and prevent the development of chronic diseases. In recent years, the number of diets based on natural foods has increased. Society has also witnessed a dietary trend that encourages the consumption of a variety and suitable amount of food in view of each person's physical and mental nature, and the consumption of food within the limits of satiety or hunger. However, the diet for longevity has not been distinctly addressed. Knowing that by 2030, the world will have one billion elderly individuals, the concept of developing a diet to optimize longevity should be the label of food production companies, specialists, medical doctors, and patients who are looking for a better life with advancing years.

The escalating incidence of age-related diseases is a medical and societal threat in countries worldwide. The rate of growth of the elderly population worldwide has seen a steep increase over the past few decades and is higher in developing than in developed countries. In addition to the demographic transition, changes in lifestyle and an increased exposure to adverse physical, chemical, and biological agents have contributed to an increase in the incidence and prevalence of chronic degenerative diseases. Humankind has faced age-related diseases and dementia since the origin of civilization. Understanding aging and old age diseases and the delay of aging are of interest to humankind, and the dream of extending life surely goes along with aging gracefully. The dream is an old one indeed, but very few things in aging research have stimulated the enthusiasm that anti-aging research has. An increased lifespan is certainly important, but it is not what interests us most; what we want to achieve is an increase in healthy life expectancy, not simply to extend the associated time of ill health.

20.1. Reducing Risk Factors for Age-Related Diseases

Twenty-first century doctors hope to help the elderly not only survive but survive well. Rather than use scarce medical resources disorder by disorder, they look to mitigate as many age-related problems as possible by dealing with the risk factors. Most of the factors are well known and can be substantially modified by relatively simple methods. Some, such as B and T cell function, relate to a progressive immune failure that will affect each of us in some way as we grow older. Other high-priority factors include the continuing change in body composition as fat increases and muscle decreases. The critical balance of testosterone and estrogen will be a factor as long as the sex hormones are present. Protecting genetic integrity is essential, but the benefits of guarding this variable in increasing the human lifespan appear to be increasing, since in the data that have been accumulated in humans so far, those achieving extremely long lives seem to portray an overall average increase in cancer susceptibility. The damage may be so intrinsic to metabolic processes that extending the maximum human lifespan may turn out to be biologically infeasible.

CHAPTER 20

Culinary Techniques for Longevity

Culinary Techniques for Longevity_Instance 2: Western culinary techniques provide quick and easy ways to transform raw produce into scrumptious meals. However, the health benefits of some protective nutrients risk being compromised by high heat exposure. Increased flavonols and reduced tannin concentrations (from apples and potatoes, respectively) show the importance of rethinking high heat handling of nutritionally-important ingredients. The anti-cancer potential of broccoli becomes a non-issue, and the increment of curcuminoid concentration in Melakan Portuguese chicken curry surprisingly contradicts the poor curcumin bioavailability odds.

Culinary Techniques for Longevity_Instance 1: Cooking techniques are essential components of the culinary arts; they transform raw ingredients into edible and flavorful meals. Culinary techniques are instrumental for health and longevity as they can lift the nutrient load from the food and heighten bioavailability of certain protective nutrients. This section features chapter-related techniques such as steaming, blanching, stir-frying, microwaving, slow-cooking, and other preparations.

21.1. Healthy Cooking Methods for Anti-Aging

Soften or mix butter, margarine or mayonnaise with vegetables. Season vegetables with herbs and spices instead of butter. Use a low-fat salad dressing or lightly drizzled olive oil on salads. Limit your intake of sugars, salt, caffeine, and manufactured foods with loose or unlisted ingredients. Eat oat bran, barley, brown rice, or grain products with at least two grams of dietary fiber per serving to protect against age-related diseases. Eat whole grain breads, such as whole wheat or rye, which are full of desirable vitamins and minerals. Use low-fat cheese and milk. Tofu is a good source of protein, calcium, and other desirable attributes of dairy foods.

Baste, steam or stir-fry foods in a small amount of vegetable oil or broth; avoid frying. Grill, broil, bake, poach or microwave foods to reduce fat and fatty acid intake. Eat a diet rich in fresh fruits and vegetables to protect against cell damage. Fresh fruits contain natural fruit sugars that energize the body and help make the perfect sweet snack. Fresh vegetables contain fiber and are low in fat, unlike snack foods. They are also low in calories and therefore a good food to include in meal plans for successful weight management. Eat a wide variety of locally grown, seasonal fruits and vegetables including dark green leafy vegetables and dried beans for fiber, vitamins, and antioxidants.

CHAPTER 21

Eating for Longevity on a Budget

If you want to eat for the long term, it completely makes sense to be frugal. And frugal doesn't have to mean depriving yourself of good taste. Quite the contrary. When it comes to cost-effectiveness, whole grains, for example, are much cheaper than paying a premium for many refined products that may not necessarily be enriched or fortified. In many cases, whole grains have been shown to be lower in calorie content per serving. Legumes are another example of the cost-benefits of eating healthfully. Rice and beans, for example, are a far healthier, cheaper, and more delicious dish than nearly any fast-food brown-bag special. Combine whole legumes with whole grains, and you have a clever and cost-effective way of providing your body with complete protein at a lower price than buying red meat or poultry. Since nuts can be sometimes pricey, just incorporate them into a healthy diet on occasion. Making your own vegetable soup is a cost-effective and delicious way of ensuring that you are indeed "soaking up" all of the benefits of vegetables. Nothing nourishes the wallet and the body when it comes down to effective eating.

The anti-aging diet truly is not expensive! Whole grains are cheap. Often, entire means of protein are less expensive than prepared ones once added together. Fresh fruits and vegetables are more expensive than they should be, but overall we can do well here. Only nuts are quite expensive and they do not have to be part of an anti-aging diet to make it work. If you can afford to eat out, you can probably afford to eat in. Meat (both fresh and frozen), poultry (both fresh and frozen), milk, cheese, yogurt, tofu, spaghetti sauce, fresh and dried legumes, whole grain pastas, brown rice, regular rice, corn meal, bulgur, and couscous. Included are potatoes, sweet potatoes, onions, tomatoes, carrots, and frozen vegetables. Also include some canned fruits, particularly if your portion size is small.

22.1. Affordable Nutrient-Rich Foods

Eggs, notably egg yolks (sorry, for those who only eat the whites), are extremely nutritious, especially when the hens have been allowed to roam around freely and eat insects, seeds, grass, and greens. As with animal liver, the nutrients provided by eggs are hardly equaled by any other food variety. Farmers market sources and small organic markets are also great places to find reasonably priced free-range eggs. Regardless of the amount of bacon, cheese, and extra virgin olive oil that you include with them, Omega 3 egg yolks scrambled with some butter, fresh herbs (such as cilantro, mint, parsley, or tarragon) and spinach or any other green you have on hand are delicious and as bright yellow as the morning sun. Aim for organic and natural foods without pesticides, toxins, or residues, and of high dietary quality. Even among those who do not have a significant budget at their disposal, to have and maintain a healthy and flexible body, as well as vibrant and radiant skin and good health, basic respected recommendations of food quality compliance wherever possible can be followed.

Beans, legumes, and lentils, boiled and then used for salads and dips, as well as fresh chicken and vegetable broths, are high in glutathione, a natural molecule so essential for the preservation of Vitamin C and E potency in the cells and a most efficient detoxifying agent activated in the liver. Animal livers, particularly the brain and kidneys, definitely may gross some people out big time, but the truth is that they are chock full of nutrients. In traditional diets, practically no part of an animal was ever wasted. Nowadays, however, they are forgotten by many people, hardly consumed, and can be found at very affordable prices at special butcher shops for paté, Belgian, Dutch, and Russian dishes. Among the internal organs, the liver is most nutritionally prolific, a great source of vital nutrients like coQ10, alpha-lipoic acid, niacin, vitamins A and C, copper, iron, and vitamins B6 and B12.

When someone says that living long and healthy is possible by eating nutrient-rich foods, the mental image that first pops up for many people is that of an exclusive gourmet menu loaded with exotic, pricey imported foods. Of course, to some extent, a bulging wallet may help, but in reality, a frugal diet is possible. You may have to do more preparation work yourself to eat the kind of meals that will nurture a healthful old age via your own home-cooked meals rather than relying all the time on ready-packed and prepared supermarket meals or eating in expensive restaurants. Not only is the nutrient content higher in simple unprocessed foods made with the best ingredients, you also avoid the chemical additives used in cheaper, ready-prepared supermarket meals.

CHAPTER 22

Ethical and Sustainable Eating for Longevity

Ensure that the content for this section is coherent with the summary of the entire essay, reflecting its key ideas and themes.

When we think about the best choices for longevity, we must also think about what is good for the planet in general, for other sentient beings, and for those who come after us. After all, many of the consequences of our food choices are not just about today. The Earth's natural resources do not generally reset overnight. If we do not eat in a sustainable way, the planet cannot sustain us indefinitely. An example of unsustainable behavior is that humans continue to dump huge amounts of pesticide into our environment to control overpopulating insect pests. We need to think in a global long-term context, and part of that is to think about eating in a more global long-term context. We must take care of the planet in order for it to take care of us. Socially conscious or ethical eating can coincide with eating for our own health and our own longevity.

23.1. The Environmental Impact of Food Choices

Guided by these core principles and the broad and diverse range of topics and issues related to enhancing human health, vitality and longevity, age-associated diseases and co-morbidities, food security and safety on a local and international scale, bestowing compassion on food animals and other non-domestic animals, animal welfare, food justice and equity, and fostering personal and societal compassion, empathy, kindness, and generosity this information provided in this chapter will address, discuss, and describe this entire spectrum of issues related to human healthy lifespan and the foods used to achieve this worthy objective. The content provided is supported by scientific evidence, especially lifetime data from the Longevity and Healthy Aging research "Cohort Study" Project. Future research on the scientific merit and effectiveness of the evidence-based dietary recommendations for health, mental vitality, and promoting Longevity are high priorities.

A high standard of diet optimization for health and longevity can only be reached by addressing a range of serious issues in the entire spectrum of on-farm and industrial food production, processing, and commercialization systems, food consumption supply chains, as well as the institutional, policy, and formal educational systems associated with these challenges. In addition to optimizing diet quality, especially for enhancing the mental and physical functionality and reducing the risks of age-related diseases for the elderly, personally health-compromised individual and population subgroups, and human longevity, the base principles that drive these dietary recommendations also generate other desirables— improved environmental well-being, national and international food security benefits, and notable compassion with respect to the well-being and welfare of food animals.

CHAPTER 23

Cultural Perspectives on Longevity and Diet

In Okinawa, the traditional Okinawan rice and vegetable dish takikomi gohan, bukubuku-cha (foaming tea) made from jasmine tea, tofu and mugwort, éirasaá and mozuku seaweed soup, among others congee. These meals that are prepared with everyday ingredients including soy, green and yellow vegetables, seaweed, sake lees, rice, tea and sesame were consumed by people of all ages on a daily basis and have no special connotations. However, with a high nutrient density and well-balanced protein, lipid, and carbohydrate content, these dishes are highly compatible with health and promote the prevention and improvement of diseases, control of stress, and extension of life expectancy. In the words of Longevity Diet proponents, the simplicity of daily life and a focus on traditional home-cooked meals cooked with tea incorporated into cuisine produces a feeling of happiness, relaxation, joy, and appreciation and contains valuable elements that contribute to vitality and a long life.

The cultural perspectives of the so-called longevity societies concerning diet revolve more around foods befitting special diets such as those consumed during certain periods or for special occasions than daily meals that promote health and longevity. Accompanying the scenes of the Longevity Diet are special meals and seasonal food festivals such as the Satsuki-kan (Fifth Month Dry Food) that are celebrated on the fifth day of the fifth month according to the old lunar calendar and the Chrysanthemum Festival held in Fukuoka City to wish for longevity. In these ancient customs, which originated in ancient China and have been handed down over generations, a variety of foods and presentations with auspicious connotations such as pine mushrooms, bamboo shoots, squid, seaweed, and ginseng are consumed as a token of appreciation for long life, good health, and continued longevity.

24.1. Traditional Diets and Longevity

The traditional diets are frequently rich in what we now identify scientifically as anti-aging vitamins, minerals, and other factors. These foods contain a unique and complex array of compounds, such as antioxidants and flavonoids. Such foods not only supply the nutrients but also produce a vitalizing, energy-rich quality in the people who consume them. Groups of people who followed traditional diets have begun to change their habits in favor of the "modern" Western diet. What happened when people transitioned from their traditional diets to Western diets? Their health started disintegrating; there was a corresponding increase in the incidence of degenerative diseases. These people enjoyed vibrant health for centuries before they adapted to the foods of Western civilization. Switching to and staying on the Western diet soon enough got them fat, made them feeble, and gave them the diseases we now link with obesity.

Traditional diets have blessed people all over the world with robust health, and faithful adherence to the dietary principles of their grandparents continues to produce the best, most consistent health results. The macronutrient (protein, carbohydrate, and fat) composition of these traditional diets varies considerably, from the largely fat-based diet in the extreme cold of the Arctic to the staple grain-based diet of the people who live in other cooler and temperate regions. These traditional diets don't stop where the energy foods (protein, fat, carbohydrate) do; they go on to include specific foods and spices that protect against the signs and symptoms of aging and help maintain the vigor of every cell, organ, and gland in our body.

CHAPTER 24

Longevity Research and Emerging Trends

There is ongoing research in the area of functional foods and nutraceuticals, including those aimed at preserving the skin, mitochondria, and the immune and cardiovascular systems. In summary, the search for novel treatments is ongoing, and nutrition is one of the most powerful strategies against aging, fighting both aging as a whole (as a result of chronic damage with accumulation of senescent cells) and environmental aging (as a result of poor-quality lifestyle choices). Since dietary intervention is responsible for prolonging the life and vitality of organisms, it represents a unique medical triumph, and one goal of the research in the field of aging is to better understand these mechanisms.

Although there is a considerable amount of data on the effects of nutrition on longevity, the process by which this occurs and the specific requirements of individual species are not yet clear. The best-known dietary intervention for extending lifespan is calorie restriction. Nutritional factors include short-chain nutritional status, antioxidants, glucose and lipid metabolism, amino acid composition of the diet, and the control of protein synthesis. In addition, markers of longevity such as nitric oxide, IGF-1, adiponectin, leptin, and the cortisol/DHEA ratio can also be altered by dietary intervention, including supplementation.

25.1. Innovations in Anti-Aging Science

The most interesting of modern research efforts start with the pace of development of biotechnology. All of a sudden, the laboratory tools and expertise needed to work on genes, cells, and proteins have rapidly become so cheap that there is a crowd of researchers, entrepreneurs, and organizations working in topics such as senolytic treatments to clear senescent cells from old people and thereby rejuvenate the old, or the age-related decline of the immune system, or the enhanced regeneration demonstrated by species such as salamanders, or indeed the natural differences in aging processes between long-lived or short-lived lineages amongst the shorter-lived mammals. The quality of the science differs, of course, but in any case all of these are just variations on themes that we know work very well - because they are practiced as a lifestyle by sizable human populations - even if little else is yet certain when it comes to the details and caveats.

One of the really interesting features of medical science today is that there are numerous approaches to the problems of degeneration, damage, and disease which are characteristic of humans as they age. The majority of these are new and barely researched, but promising. They are not poking at the symptoms of aging, they are poking at the root causes. We can largely absent ourselves from most of the advances, however, given that it is already well known that a calorie restriction mimetic drug like metformin, acting as a very subtle metabolic signal of calorie restriction, can slow aging and significantly reduce age-related disease and mortality in most people.

CHAPTER 25

Practical Tips for Incorporating Longevity Principles

Remember, no one can do everything that is good for her or him all at once. It is important to realize that just making the effort to change one bad habit, or incorporate one new good habit would make a difference. Changes will make a difference. It may take longer to see a change, but that should not be an excuse for indifference on your part. At this stage, our goals should be to prevent illness, preserve as much body function as possible, and to prevent disability. Being healthy and having a high quality of life in these years should remain our primary objective. A very active role in your own health care will improve the quality of your life and length of survival. Individuals are quickly taking a leading role in their own health care under the principles of an anti-aging lifestyle. This means participating in making good health a way of life.

There is no cookie-cutter approach; we are each different and have different requirements. Still, there are general rules that we can all follow, principles that have stood the test of time and are endorsed by the major health organizations. Following an anti-aging lifestyle is not about following rules, it is a way of life. It is a practice through which we create habits that will decrease our likelihood of having long-term chronic diseases so that we can have a full active life free of infirmities, for as long as the good Lord intended for us. Dr. Franklin Beers' guidelines are simple, they are inclusive. Eating well, limiting bad habits and taking the "whole" person into account, are the three underlying principles of this lifestyle that Dr. Beers has put into practice in his own lifestyle.

26.1. Simple Strategies for Long-Term Health

Refined carbohydrates skyrocket blood sugar, increase insulin release, and result in the formation of those blood vessel-damaging free radicals; in contrast, complex carbohydrates, which are digested more slowly, lead to a slower, more even rise in blood sugar and the formation of fewer free radicals. Getting sufficient vitamin E, often labeled the anti-aging vitamin, is as easy as taking a walk and consuming a diet that includes sprouted wheat germ, almonds, sunflower seeds, pumpkin seeds, and flaxseeds, and sweet potatoes, whole grains, avocados, stone fruits, berries, and papayas. Vitamin E decreases the risk for heart disease, dementia, Alzheimer's disease, and Parkinson's disease while interfering with the lipid oxidation steps in the production of those pesky age-necrotizing free radicals. Don't worry about the dietary cholesterol in the overcrowded category of items to worry about; the cholesterol found in food is not what causes cardiovascular disease. In addition, moderate alcohol intake is associated with a decreased risk of heart disease, cancer, and diabetes, and the overall death rates. Women: no more than one drink per day; men: no more than two drinks per day.

We know that aging involves wear and tear on the cellular and molecular level. It's as if we "rust" like spoons and cars left unprotected too long. So simple strategies for slapping on a metaphorical coat of antioxidant protection from the everyday blast of free radicals are well worth the effort. Eat more fruits and vegetables - especially leafy, green vegetables and deeply pigmented ones. It's now proven that their high antioxidant content benefits your cells, tissues, and organs in general and your brain in particular. The beta carotene in carrots and the lutein in spinach and kale, for example, significantly reduce the risk of cataracts and age-related macular degeneration, the major causes of vision impairment in the elderly. Vegetables high in beta carotene and vitamin C, such as sweet potatoes and oranges, protect your respiratory system and lungs. And the vitamin C in many of the vegetables has antioxidant effects that bolster your immune function. Eat more whole grains and legumes. The focus on anti-aging is predominantly on two very common diseases - cancer and heart disease. Epidemiological studies confirm that a diet high in fiber, particularly from whole grains and legumes, is the gold standard for reducing colon cancer risk. Research linking whole grains and nuts with a decreased risk of diabetes and heart disease is more controversial but still intriguing.

CHAPTER 26

Conclusion and Future Directions

To achieve such health benefits, it is crucial to find simple and reproducible ways to prolong the healthy period of life. Although many molecules and signaling pathways have been proposed to delay aging, safe and robust methods that can be used by any lay person still need to be identified. For centuries, combinations of diet and specific food components have been known to influence lifespan in various organisms, including mammals. Under this context, the design of an "anti-aging diet" appears to be a feasible and pragmatic approach to delay the time of onset of age-related diseases and increase the health span of the general human population.

Nutrition strategies that optimize health and reduce the risk of developing various diseases are vital for good public health, especially in developed societies in which the lack of high physical workload has led to a high prevalence of metabolic disorders (obesity, diabetes, liver steatosis, etc.). On the other hand, life expectancy has increased, and contemporary science recognized the aging process itself as a primary risk factor for all kinds of age-related diseases. If we can slow the rate of aging and extend the period of healthy aging (health span), both individual people and society could have significant benefits. Reduction of the aging process in various model organisms has given researchers better insight into the hallmarks and molecular components of the aging process. Using this knowledge to slow the rate of human aging has become a much more targeted and realistic goal.

27.1. Summary of Key Takeaways

Research supports a diet composed of plentiful fruits, vegetables, and lean protein, primarily from unsaturated fats found in plant sources which potentially protect us from numerous chronic health risks, including DNA damage, gene instability, and chronic inflammation. Additionally, a healthy eating plan helps protect against cellular aging. Avoiding processed meats, fast food, soft drinks, tobacco in any form, pitch black coffee, and an overabundance of unhealthy fats, especially those of animal origin, is just as important as adding fruits, vegetables, whole grains, healthy protein, and dairy to our diet, due to their powerful disease prevention potential. Eat with purpose, saving unhealthy treats as a reward for prudent eating habits. Create a conducive and intentional dietary future by carefully choosing what and how much we eat right now.

The anti-aging diet includes a variety of colorful vegetables, whole fresh fruits, lean protein, fat-free dairy products, predominantly plant-based unsaturated fats, and a limited amount of junk food. Colorful fresh produce provides nutrients that may prevent and even reverse skin aging. The protein fraction of the anti-aging diet includes fish, poultry, legumes, nonfat milk and yogurt, and eggs for healthy building functions. Unsaturated fats derived from plant sources are another crucial part of the anti-aging diet, as they offer a collection of vitamins and fatty acids that reinforce both cellular and whole-body functions. The anti-aging diet is one of the most research-based nutrition plans currently available, supporting cellular healing, DNA repair and gene protection, in addition to the prevention and slowing of illness and disease throughout life.

Milton Keynes UK
Ingram Content Group UK Ltd.
UKHW040938081224
452111UK00011B/231